SUGAR DETOX FOR BEGINNERS

21-DAY MEAL PLAN

BY NATASHA BROWN

Presented by French Number Publishing
French Number Publishing is an independent publishing house headquartered in Paris, France with offices in North America, Europe, and Asia.
FN⁹ is committed to connect the most promising writers to readers from all around the world. Together we aim to explore the most challenging issues on a large variety of topics that are of interest to the modern society.

FREE DOWNLOAD

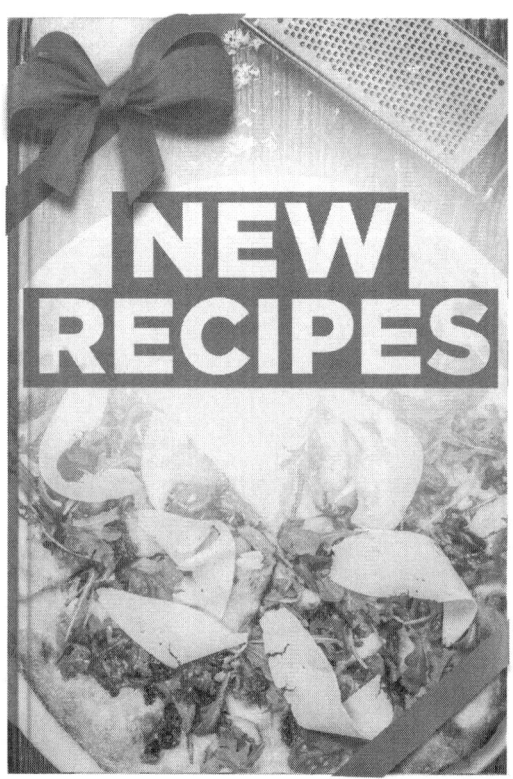

YOUR FREE GIFT!
GET MORE FREE RECIPES IN 1 CLICK!

GET YOUR FREE RECIPES HERE:

www.frenchnumber.net/detox21

INTRODUCTION

DAY 1

DAY 2

DAY 3

DAY 4

DAY 5

DAY 6

DAY 7

DAY 8

DAY 9

DAY 10

DAY 11

DAY 12

DAY 13

DAY 14

DAY 15

DAY 16

INTRODUCTION

HOW SUGAR GOT ITS BAD REP...

In order to properly and effectively detox from "Bad" sugar, it is necessary to first understand what exactly sugar is, why your body needs it and why there are "Good" sugars and "Bad" sugars.

Basically, the three types of carbohydrates found in the human diet (sugar, starch and fiber) are all sugar. Simple sugars consist of one or two molecules of sugar, start to break down in the mouth, and because they are so quickly introduced to the bloodstream, cause a spike in blood sugar and make us feel temporarily energetic, followed soon after by a crash. Think of how you feel 15 minutes after eating that mid-afternoon candy bar and sugar-laced coffee, and you get the picture. Starch and fiber, on the other hand, are complex sugars because they are made from three to hundreds of sugar molecules, take longer to digest, enter the bloodstream more slowly and give us a more even, sustained form of energy.

Energy is good. Hence, naturally occurring sugar found in fruits, vegetables, beans, nuts and whole grains, eaten in moderation, is "Good" sugar. Sugar, when accompanied by vitamins, minerals, protein, phytochemicals and fiber, which slows down the absorption of sugar in the bloodstream, equals a steady, consistent energy for our bodies to consume and run well on. However, when sugar is gratuitously added to food during processing, cooking or at the table, it becomes a source of extra calories with no nutritional value or fiber to slow the energy down. This "added" sugar is the "Bad" sugar that coats ALL sugar with a bad reputation. This book is filled with recipes designed to eliminate and detox "Bad" sugars from your diet and body in under a month!

So why is sugar added to food if it's such a bad thing? Primarily, sugar is a cheap, effective flavor enhancer. It boosts and amplifies the taste and texture of foods, ranging from desserts and snacks to more surprising foods, such as soup, bread and most shocking of all, Low and FAT-FREE foods like yoghurt and frozen dinners!

An even more insidious "benefit" of adding sugar to food, is its addictive quality. Basically, the addition of simple sugars, i.e., easily broken-down and digested sugars into foods, starts a vicious cycle of energy spikes and crashes which result in cravings for more and more of this quick-fix energy. Ironically, the very foods chosen by people trying to lose extra weight end up packing the pounds on, as well as flooding the body and blood with tons of sugary energy that can't be processed quickly enough. The body has to do something with the excess, so it stores this energy, in the form of FAT. Eventually, this continuous onslaught of sugar throws entire systems of the body off, and like the sludge of old oil in a car, our bodies become increasingly clogged up and less able to function at optimal capacity.

THE BENEFITS OF SUGAR DETOX:

The following list of benefits gained when you embark on a 21 or 10-day "bad" sugar detox are not, as you will discover, limited to your general health. Eliminating foods that contain added sugar will have a profound impact on many levels of your life!

- Weight Loss: Eating whole vs. "processed" foods with added sugar in moderation aids in better digestion, elimination and weight control
- Cost Savings: Eating foods found on "the edges" of a grocery store, i.e., fresh produce, meat, fish and whole grains, rather than "convenience" foods found in the frozen aisle, can lower food bills.
- Positive Role Modeling: Inspire your family, kids and friends to break the "Bad" sugar habit, and influence future generations!
- Increase "Real" Energy: When you eat whole foods with natural sugar, you are controlling your source of healthy, consistent and even energy intake.
- Eliminate Cravings: Stop the vicious cycle of ingesting junk food, experiencing energy spikes and crashes and repeating this negative behavior.
- Streamline your Grocery List: Buying and consuming whole foods and ingredients for sugar detox recipes will simplify your shopping.

- Stop Feeling Tired: Because of the energy highs and lows of added sugar, you end up feeling sleepy and sluggish in the middle of the day.
- Regulate Digestion: Consuming meals made up of whole foods increases fiber intake and aids in digestion and elimination.
- Clearer Skin: Unclog your body inside and out!
- Gain a "Happy" Tummy: Detoxing "Bad" sugar can help eliminate bloating, gas and nausea.
- Even out Mood Swings: Sugar spikes can result in increased anxiety. Sugar crashes can result in increased depression. Sugar detox can help control both.
- Increased Mental Clarity: If you are controlling anxiety and depression, you'll have more time to think clearly.
- Sugar Awareness: Detoxing necessitates reading the ingredient panels in everything you purchase and eat. You will become increasingly aware of all the surprising places sugar lurks.
- Improved Sleep: It stands to reason if your stomach is more settled and your energy is more consistent you will end up sleeping longer and deeper.
- •Adding Diversity to your Diet: When you detox from added sugar, you will end up having to eliminate many old standbys in your diet. The good news is you will discover new whole food taste treats you would never have tried.

TWENTY ONE OR TEN DAY MEAL PLAN OPTIONS:

I have published 2 books on sugar detox: a 21 day-option, based on the well-known theory that it takes 3 weeks to develop a new habit and fully commit to it; and a 10-day option for people who want faster results and are willing to experience more intense withdrawal symptoms. These options are both included because people are motivated by and respond to varied experiences. Rather than a "one-size-fits-all" approach, you will be given two time frames in which to detox.

21-day Habit Modification Plans work on the assumption that a three-week time frame gives your body and mind a generous amount of time to adjust to positive change without undue stress or deprivation. It's also a lot more reasonable to tell yourself that you can cut out the offending habit, or in this case, food source for 21 days, rather than go cold turkey and declare that you will NEVER eat sugar again for the rest of your life. After the initial 21 day period, your body and mind have had ample time to recalibrate to life without added sugar; cravings have gradually and easily been eliminated and you have a three week period of success to look back upon and continue to motivate yourself as you look forward to a "Good" sugar future. 21 days also give you time to honestly reflect upon how you've felt in the past in comparison to how you are feeling as you detox from added "bad" sugar. This type of observation and reflection resonates well with people who require gradual transitions and more time to acclimate to change, without diminishing the positive results.

The 10-day meal plan was designed for people who are motivated by "jumping into the deep end" and who become disengaged or unmotivated by a process or plan that takes too much time. This more intense program are for those of you who are frankly sick and tired of feeling sick and tired and want to experience faster results, including the effects of a more sudden withdrawal from added sugar. People are different and the discomfort of sudden withdrawal that might discourage people drawn to the 21-day option actually motivates other people who look at these physical symptoms as concrete proof that "Bad" sugar has had such a profound effect on their well-being!

Whoever you are and whether you opted for the 21 or 10-day meal plan, both have been carefully designed to give you positive results without complicated instructions, hard-to-find ingredients and time consuming recipes. Both offer a clear, detailed approach to eliminating "Bad" added sugar from your diet by introducing delicious recipes prepared with healthful whole food ingredients

THE "BAD" SUGAR DETOX MISSION

Sugar Detox was well-explained in by David Zinczenko who continues his twenty-year mission to help people live their happiest and healthiest lives, uncovering revolutionary new research that explains why you can't lose weight – and shows that it's not your fault! The true culprit is sugar – specifically added sugars – which food manufacturers sneak into almost everything we eat, from bread to cold cuts to yoghurt, peanut butter, pizza, and even "health foods".

Do you ever watch old movies or TV shows and watch in resentful wonder as slim, attractive all American families sit down to eat huge home-cooked meals, complete with desserts? What happened? It doesn't make sense, that 50 years later, with all of our education, scientific and technological advances and understanding about the benefit of proper nutrition and exercise we have become a nation full of obesity, diabetes and stress-related disease!

The research has been conducted and compiled and the results clearly show that a major culprit of our increasingly unhealthy society is the addition of sugar to almost EVERY processed food we buy and consume today!

According to the American Heart Association (AHA) the maximum amount of added sugar you should eat a day for men is 9 tsp, and for women 6 tsp. With that in mind, here are just a few examples of tsp of added sugar in one serving of processed foods:

- One can of regular soda: 8 tsp sugar
- One chocolate bar: 5.75 tsp of sugar
- Froot Loops cereal: 10.5 tsp of sugar
- ½ cup pasta sauce: 3 tsp of sugar
- One serving instant oatmeal: between 3 and 4 tsp of sugar
- 1 tablespoon of Ketchup: 1 tsp of sugar

From the examples above, it's easy to see how you could exceed your daily recommended allowance in one snack or a few ingredients in a typical meal.

Sugar is added to foods for many reasons; none of which are to benefit your wellbeing. It is added to baked goods as a preservative to keep them fresher longer, to keep jellies and jams from spoiling, to aid in the fermentation process in bread and alcohol and to improve the color of foods and drinks!

Another sneaky way that sugar is added to your foods, especially those you may be buying because they are "healthy" and/or "organic" and "natural", is by listing it by other names, such as; agave syrup, brown sugar, corn sweetener and corn syrup, fructose, glucose, honey, malt syrup, raw sugar or molasses.

No matter what it's added to or what it's called, in the fight against added sugar, it sometimes feels as if you simply can't win for losing. How can you be blamed for gaining weight and jeopardizing your health when you have been consuming food and drink that has been literally "laced" with tons of added sugar?

This book has been conceived and written as a concrete weapon in the battle of added "Bad" sugar. It is full of healthy, delicious recipes that use whole food ingredients free from added sugar and empty calories. By simply following the 21 or 10 day meal plans, you will transform your diet from one filled with hidden "bad" sugar, to a nutritionally dense and filling menu of meals composed of foods bursting with vitamins, minerals, and "good" sugar that will give you authentic energy, allowing you to experience renewed vigor and a sense of balanced well-being.

Armed with nutritionally sound knowledge you will view the typical supermarket with clear, open eyes. As you shop, you will bypass many old favorites and menu standbys, now that you understand how unhealthy they are for you and your loved ones. Instead you will choose simpler, whole foods with no added ingredients, secure in the knowledge that you know EXACTLY what you are putting in your recipes and, ultimately, into your body.

So often nowadays you read about how fat, lazy and inactive American adults and their children are. Yet, the media is crammed with the latest health and fitness crazes and billions of dollars are spent every year on sports equipment, gym memberships, diet programs and food plans. You can't help but wonder why none of this incredible effort, time and money isn't improving the statistics. Again, it comes down to the irrefutable fact, that we are literally eating our weight in added sugar and empty calories. And the destruction doesn't stop there. Frighteningly, the more of this nutritionally bankrupt food we consume; the more we crave it, ingesting it in larger and larger quantities, even when it has been marketed to us as "low" or "no-fat"! In any other environment, this hypocrisy would be viewed as a criminal offense and punished as a highly illegal and immoral act. Yet, when it comes to our health, our very well-being, we continue to consume this subtle but devastating poison.

The health benefits of eating whole foods and "good" sugars are only part of the good news. Once you are firmly positioned on the road to physical good health, your mental and emotional wellbeing will improve as well. As you regain energy and vigor you will be able to enjoy life and accomplish goals you had once given up as impossibilities. Your economic health will also improve, as you rely less on processed, convenience foods and meals, and more on freshly prepared ingredients. Your tastes will evolve too and you will find yourself reaching into the fruit bowl rather than scrambling for extra cash to fund the empty calories found in a vending machine, coffee shop or fast food restaurant.

It all comes down to the difference between living to eat and eating to live. The possibility that we have been sold, along with added "Bad" sugar, the empty promise that if you eat this processed, "convenience" food, you will somehow be given more time to enjoy your life, fuelled by the temporary jolt of sweetened energy is one we must face down once and for all before it defeats our health and happiness. Rather, if we relearn to eat the foods nature has always provided us, free from added sugar, we can detox ourselves from an addictive, unnecessary ingredient in a relatively short period of time. When you consider it took years and years of eating poorly to get us to such a perilous state of health, ten or twenty one days is a mere blip on the timeline of life!

Ending any sort of food addiction can be a daunting, even overwhelming challenge. Unlike smoking, or gambling or most any other addiction, you simply cannot quit food. This book has been written with that knowledge constantly in mind. Through the 21 or 10-day meal plans, you will be able to eliminate the one element; added "Bad" sugar, which has tainted the food you have been eating. Once the added sugar has been eliminated and healthy whole food sources with natural "good" sugar have replaced it, you will have the time you personally require, be it 21 or 10 days, to acclimate yourself to the benefits of this one change as well as to experience the positive changes you will soon see in your physical health, mental clarity and outlook, and continued general well-being. Food is not the enemy. Naturally occurring "Good" sugar founds in fruits, vegetables, protein, beans, and whole grains isn't either. Added "Bad" sugar, introduced to our food sources to falsely enhance flavor, preservation, aesthetic appeal, economic viability and an addictive nature is the true enemy. A needless, sense-less enemy that when eradicated will open our minds and bodies to the potential gift of true, lasting health. All you need is the desire to rid yourself of an unconscious, unhealthy habit. This book and its delicious 21 or 10-day meal plans will provide the rest of the solution!

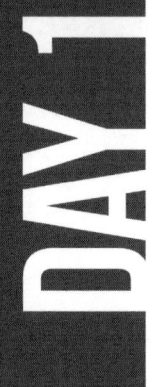

SPINACH PANCAKES

/ SERVES 4 / PREPARATION TIME 10 MIN. / COOKINGTIME 10 MIN. /

INGREDIENTS

1	pack of chopped spinach (Frozen) Preferably 16 oz.
1	finely chopped onion (Medium sized)
¼	cup parsley (chopped)
1	tbsp minced garlic
3	medium to large eggs
1	tbsp kosher salt
½	tbsp black pepper (for taste)
¼	cup cheese (Parmesan)
2	tbsp olive oil (For the purpose of frying)

NUTRITION PER SERVING

CALORIES — 145   PROTEIN — 20   FIBER — 5
SUGARS — 2   FAT — 28

INSTRUCTIONS

1. Use a pan or a microwave to boil the spinach over medium heat.

2. By pressing hard on the spinach, drain the excess water using a kitchen towel.

3. Mix the spinach, parsley, onion and the garlic in a medium to large sized bowl.

4. On the other end, using the salt and the pepper, finely whisk the eggs and add it to the spinach mixture along with the healthy Parmesan cheese. Mix the ingredients thoroughly using a spatula.

5. Heat the olive oil (1 tbsp) in two large non-stick skillets over medium to high heat. In order to evenly coat, you could brush throughout the griddle.

6. Employ an ice cream scoop to take the mixture out and press down to flatten the mixture while continuing to cook for good 4 minutes until it turns brown and crisp.

7. Gently drain the mixture on the paper towel before you serve.

TIP
To make evenly shaped muffins, use a spring-loaded ice-cream scoop, which could assist in better distribution among cups.

SAUTEED LION'S MANE MUSHROOM

/ SERVES 1 / PREPARATION TIME 5 MIN. / COOKINGTIME 5 MIN. /

INGREDIENTS

1 tbsp olive oil (extra virgin)
1-2 cups sliced mushroom
2 tbsp thyme
Pinch of sea salt (to taste)
Pinch of ground pepper (to taste)

NUTRITION PER SERVING

CALORIES — 25   PROTEIN — 3   FIBER — 5
SUGARS — 1   FAT — 0

INSTRUCTIONS

1. Over a non-sticky skillet, heat the extra virgin olive oil over medium heat.

2. Introduce sliced mushrooms to the pan, and sprinkle a little salt and pepper as per your convenience.

3. Keep stirring for the next 3 minutes until the mixture turns golden brown in color.

4. Complete the recipe with a little addition of thyme and take it off the heat to serve.

CILANTRO LIME SHRIMP WITH ZUCCHINI NOODLES

/ SERVES 4 / PREPARATION TIME 10 MIN. / COOKINGTIME 15 MIN. /

INGREDIENTS

2	tbsp butter
1	pound of shelled jumbo shrimp
4	finely chopped garlic cloves
1	pinch red pepper flakes
¼	cup white wine or chicken broth or shrimp broth or vegetable broth
2	tbsp lime juice
3	medium sized finely chopped noodles like zucchini
1	tbsp lime zest
2	tbsp chopped cilantro

Salt and pepper to taste

NUTRITION PER SERVING

CALORIES — 212   PROTEIN — 25   FIBER — 2
SUGARS — 5   FAT — 8

INSTRUCTIONS

1. Over medium to high heat, melt the butter in a pan until it starts frothing.

2. Add the shrimp followed by cooking for 2 minutes, flipping, bringing in the garlic and red pepper flakes (optional) and cook the ingredients for 1 more minute before putting the shrimp aside.

3. Introduce the white wine and lime juice to the pan, deglaze it and boil the ingredients for the next 2 minutes.

4. Add the zucchini noodles and cook until they get delicate and soft, for about 2 minutes, before dressing the ingredients with salt and pepper while adding the shrimp, lime zest and cilantro, tossing everything and removing from the heat.

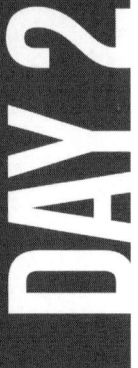

SAUTED CHICKEN MUSHROOM OMLETTE

/ SERVES 4 / PREPARATION TIME 15 MIN. / COOKINGTIME 5 MIN. /

INGREDIENTS

An egg along with **3** egg whites

1 tbsp Parmesan cheese

1 tbsp cheddar cheese (shredded)

¼ tbsp sea salt (for taste)

⅓ tbsp red pepper flakes (crushed)

⅓ tbsp garlic powder

⅓ tbsp ground pepper

½ cup mushrooms (sliced)

2 tbsp green peppers (finely chopped)

1 tbsp onion (finely chopped)

½ tbsp olive oil

A cup of chicken sausage cut into slices

NUTRITION PER SERVING

CALORIES — 255.2   PROTEIN — 33.4   FIBER — 2.3

SUGARS — 1.4   FAT — 10.3

INSTRUCTIONS

1. Beat the egg and egg whites in a small bowl.
2. Mix the cheeses well, add salt, pepper flakes, garlic powder and pepper, and place it aside.
3. Sauté the mushrooms, green pepper and onions in an 8-inch non-sticky skillet for up to 5 minutes or until it gets tender.
4. Add chicken sausage while continuing to cook and stir until the chicken gets warm.
5. Introduce the egg mixture.
6. Once the eggs set underneath, lift the edges while allowing the uncooked portion to smoothly flow underneath.
7. Chop into fine wedges and serve immediately.

TIP
The omelette's preparation consists of cubes of strips of meat cooked on skewers and served with spicy peanut sauce.

CAULIFLOWER AGRODOLCE

/ SERVES 8 / PREPARATION TIME 10 MIN. / COOKINGTIME 20 MIN. /

INGREDIENTS

2	cauliflower heads cut into florets
4	cups of onions
6	Finely sliced garlic cloves
2	tbsp extra virgin olive oil
1	cup wine vinegar
½	cup of parsley
6	tbsp of capers (optional)

Sea salt and pepper to taste

NUTRITION PER SERVING

CALORIES — 125   PROTEIN — 4   FIBER — 6

SUGARS — 1   FAT — 5

INSTRUCTIONS

1. Finely blanch the head and florets of the cauliflower for 5 minutes and set it to one side.

2. Gently stir the onions together with the garlic in olive oil until and they become soft and tender, for about two minutes.

3. Introduce the vinegar slowly and simmer it for about 5 minutes.

4. Combine all the ingredients and add cauliflower to it while cooking it for the next 10 minutes.

5. Add salt and pepper as per your convenience and cook for the next 2 minutes.

6. Garnish with parsley and add capers for extra saltiness.

SPICY HONEY GARLIC SALMON IN FOIL

/ SERVES 4 / PREPARATION TIME 5 MIN. / COOKINGTIME 25 MIN. /

INGREDIENTS

About **5** ounces of salmon fillets

Sesame seeds

Coriander leaves (Finely chopped)

For sauce:

2 tbsp lemon juice

1 tbsp Dijon mustard

1 tbsp honey

4 tbsp sodium soy sauce

2 tbsp rice vinegar

1 tbsp ginger

Freshly grated sriracha about **1** tbsp

1 tsp. red chilli flakes

1 tsp. garlic

3 minced cloves oregano

¼ tsp. kosher salt to taste

Freshly ground black pepper to taste

2 tbsp sesame oil

1 lime zest

NUTRITION PER SERVING

CALORIES — 230   PROTEIN — 22   FIBER — 0
SUGARS — 8   FAT — 11

 ## INSTRUCTIONS

1. Preheat oven to 375 degrees F.
2. Nicely crease the baking sheet using foil.
3. Dry the salmons using a paper towel.
4. Whip the ingredients in a small bowl, under the sauce.
5. Put the salmon into the sauce and place them in the lined baking sheet.
6. Carefully spoon the leftover mixture over the salmon.
7. In order to seal the pack, fold the sides of the foil over the salmon and shield it completely.
8. Now place the sealed packs into the microwave and bake for about 15- 20 minutes until they are cooked through.
9. Open the packed and roast them for about 2 -3 minutes for it to get caramelized and slightly cauterized.
10. Serve hot by finely decorating with chopped coriander leaves and sesame seeds.

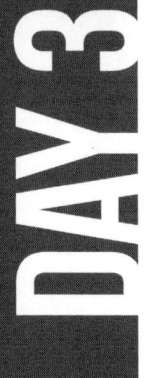

DAY 3

OAT HONEY CRUMBLE

/ SERVES 1 / PREPARATION TIME 10 MIN. / COOKINGTIME 1 HOUR /

INGREDIENTS

	A cup of honey
	A cup of rolled oats
	A cup of -purpose flour
½	cup melted butter
3	cups apples (finely peeled and chopped)
2	tbsp ground cinnamon

NUTRITION PER SERVING

CALORIES — 150   PROTEIN — 4   FIBER — 0
SUGARS — 1.6   FAT — 6

INSTRUCTIONS

1. Preheat oven to 350 degrees F and gently grease the square pan (8 inch).

2. Combine honey, oats, flour and butter in a large bowl and continue to stir and mix until the mixture becomes crumbly.

3. Keep almost half of crumb mixture in a pan and spread the apples evenly over the mixture.

4. Sprinkle cinnamon over the mixture and you could additionally top with remaining crumb mixture.

5. Move on to baking the mixture for 40 to 45 minutes in the preheated oven until it turns golden brown.

TIP
Use a measuring cup or sturdy glass to assist in pressing down oats before baking. This will work wonders to help ensuring the bars hold their shape after cutting.

ROASTED POTATOS AND DILL

/ SERVES 8 / PREPARATION TIME 10 MIN. / COOKINGTIME 15 MIN. /

INGREDIENTS

1 pound of potatoes
2 tbsp extra virgin olive oil
Sea salt and pepper (to taste)
Fresh dill

NUTRITION PER SERVING

CALORIES — 250   PROTEIN — 3   FIBER — 3
SUGARS — 1.2   FAT — 7

INSTRUCTIONS

1. Preheat the microwave to 450°F and keep the potatoes in a medium to large roasting pan and toss it with extra virgin olive oil, salt and pepper to coat it evenly.

2. Place the potatoes in such a way that they create a single layer in order to be cooked uniformly.

3. Bake for the next 15-20 minutes while stirring occasionally.

4. Finally, dress it with handful of dill to serve immediately.

QUINOA AND CUCUMBER NOODLES SALAD WITH AVOCADO DRESSING

/ SERVES 1 / PREPARATION TIME 5 MIN. / COOKINGTIME 5 MIN. /

 ## INGREDIENTS

⅓   cup spiralised cucumber
⅓   cup chopped tomatoes
¼   cup avocado
¼   cup red onion
⅓   cup cooked quinoa
½   tbsp chopped parsley
FOR THE DRESSING:
¼   tbsp avocado
½   tbsp white wine vinegar
¼   tbsp lime juice
⅕   tbsp Single Meal
    Salt to taste
    Pepper to taste
    Olive oil to taste

NUTRITION PER SERVING

CALORIES — 108.8   PROTEIN — 2.5   FIBER — 1.6
SUGARS — 1.5   FAT — 5.6

INSTRUCTIONS

The salad:

1. Mix together cucumber, parsley, avocado, onion, tomato and the quinoa in a small bowl.

The dressing:

1. Merge together avocado, lemon juice, vinegar salt and pepper in a blender.
2. Carry on until smooth and creamy.
3. Bring in olive oil gradually unless and until just combined.
4. Transfer to a jar and drizzle over the salad before serving.

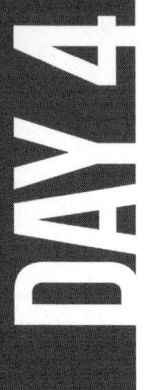

BREAKFAST SALAD (OLIVE EGG SALAD)

/ SERVES 1 BOWL / PREPARATION TIME 5 MIN. / COOKINGTIME O MIN. /

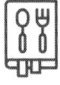

INGREDIENTS

3 tbsp dressing of miracle whip
2 tbsp brown mustard
4 finely cooked eggs (finely chopped)
6-7 green olives (pimento-stuffed)
21 wheat crackers (halved and woven)

NUTRITION PER SERVING

CALORIES — 265.1   PROTEIN — 12.7   FIBER — 0
SUGARS — 0.6   FAT — 19.5

INSTRUCTIONS

1. You could start by mixing the entire miracle whip dressing with the brown mustard in a medium to large bowl.

2. Add eggs and olives to the mixture and mix them thoroughly.

3. Finally, serve with crackers.

LEMON GINGER ROASTED CHICKEN

/ SERVES 4 / PREPARATION TIME 15 MIN. / COOKINGTIME 1 HOUR /

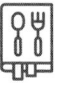

INGREDIENTS

	Whole roasted chicken (3Pounds)
2½	lemons
¼	cup lemon juice
2	tbsp lemon's zest
1	tbsp extra virgin olive oil
3	finely mashed cloves of garlic
2-3	tbsp ginger
	Small quantity of rosemary
	Sea salt and pepper to taste

NUTRITION PER SERVING

CALORIES — 194.2   PROTEIN — 34.7   FIBER — 0.2

SUGARS — 1.0   FAT — 3.0

INSTRUCTIONS

1. Preheat the oven to 400°F.
2. Remove the roasted chicken after washing it and place it within a baking pan.
3. Merge the lemon zest with the ¼ cup of lemon juice and add the mixture with a few drizzles of olive oil, salt and pepper.
4. Combine the mixture with the mashed garlic, and then pulverize for about 2-3 tbsp of ginger and mix them thoroughly.
5. Pour it over the chicken.
6. Remove the rosemary leaves and put them upon the chicken, which should be left to roast for another 1-½ hours.

SLOW COOKER WHOLE CAULIFLOWER CURRY AND CASHEW

/ SERVES 4 / PREPARATION TIME 10 MIN. / COOKINGTIME 5 HOURS /

INGREDIENTS

1	large cauliflower leaves and stems trimmed
1	red pepper, seeded and thinly sliced
2	small potatoes (we used red), quartered
½	onion, chopped
2	garlic cloves, sliced
	Toasted cashews, chopped
	Cilantro, for garnish
	The curry sauce:
2	cups vegetable broth
2	cups unsweetened coconut milk
2	tbsp yellow curry powder
1	tsp. cumin
½	tsp. cayenne pepper (to taste)

NUTRITION PER SERVING

CALORIES — 205.6   PROTEIN — 4.5   FIBER — 6.0

SUGARS — 1.2   FAT — 6.5

INSTRUCTIONS

1. Mix together the red peppers, whole cauliflower, potatoes, red peppers, garlic and onions within the slow cooker.

2. The vegetable broth, cumin, curry powder, and cayenne pepper must be whisked together in a medium to large bowl.

3. Shift this mixture into the slow cooker and mix well in order to coat cauliflower and veggies.

4. Cover the slow cooker and cook the ingredients on high for up to 3 hours. The cauliflower and other veggies will be tender way before this point, and continues to get tender as it sits.

5. Stir in coconut milk 10-15 minutes before serving.

6. Adjust the dressing with salt and pepper to serve warm.

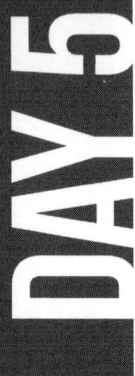

FRESH FRUIT MUSELI

/ SERVES 1 / PREPARATION TIME 5 MIN. / COOKINGTIME 0 MIN. /

INGREDIENTS

1 red apple (cored and chopped)
1 yellow apple (cored and chopped)
2 pears – (cored and chopped)
apple juice (75 ml)
1 lush green lemon
2-3 fresh strawberries
rolled oats (75 grams)
1-2 tbsp honey
yoghurt (250 ml)
2 tbsp almonds (diced)
2 tbsp raisins
1 tbsp jiggery (finely grated)

NUTRITION PER SERVING

CALORIES — 289   PROTEIN — 8.24   FIBER — 6.2
SUGARS — 4.35   FAT — 4.16

INSTRUCTIONS

1. Mix the apples and the pears in a medium pan.
2. Sprinkle the mixture to moisten it with the apple and lemon juice.
3. Mix the oats, raisins and honey in the mixture and stir well.
4. Introduce yoghurt and all other ingredients with jiggery being an exception.
5. Cover the mixture and leave it to chill.
6. Serve the muesli breakfast sprinkled with grated jiggery.

STEAMED BROCCOLI WITH KALMATA OLIVES

/ SERVES 8 / PREPARATION TIME 5 MIN. / COOKINGTIME 10 MIN. /

INGREDIENTS

Freshly cleaned
and trimmed broccoli florets (1 pound)

1 tbsp extra virgin olive oil

1 finely minced garlic clove

1 lemon

12-15 Kalamata olives chopped in half

Pepper and sea salt, to taste

NUTRITION PER SERVING

CALORIES — 74.5   PROTEIN — 3.0   FIBER — 3.3

SUGARS — 0.7   FAT — 5.1

INSTRUCTIONS

1. Keep the broccoli florets in a steamer basket. Boil the water in a covered pot, followed by cooking broccoli so that it gets crisp, for about 5 minutes.

2. Take the broccoli and place in a bowl.

3. Meanwhile, heat the olive oil in a pan over medium to high heat.

4. Introduce the olives and garlic to the pan while stirring the mixture for about 1 minute.

5. Next, introduce the lemon juice, broccoli, and pepper to the pan and check if you need any more salt or pepper..

6. Mix well to serve fresh.

TIPS
You could tightly wrap ingredients and freeze them for up to
2 months. Just about 25 minutes before serving, heat oven to 350°.

TURMERIC, CARROT AND RED LENTIL STEW

/ SERVES 6-8 / PREPARATION TIME 15 MIN. / COOKINGTIME 45 MIN. /

INGREDIENTS

3	tbsp olive oil
1	large onion, roughly chopped
4	minced garlic cloves
2	in. piece of ginger, grated or minced
1	lb. carrots chopped
1	lb. squash or pumpkin, roughly chopped
1	small bunch marjoram, tied with cooking twine
4	bay leaves
2	quarts organic vegetable or chicken broth
1½	cups red lentil
1½	tbsp ground turmeric
1	tsp. coriander
1	tbsp zatar
2	tbsp sumac
¼	tbsp cumin
⅛	tbsp cayenne
3	tbsp tamarin
5	stalks of kale, de-stemmed and torn
	Sea salt to taste
	Freshly ground pepper
	Sour cream or yogurt to serve, optional

NUTRITION PER SERVING

CALORIES — 335   PROTEIN — 20   FIBER — 23
SUGARS — 4.8   FAT — 4

 ## INSTRUCTIONS

1. Add olive oil, garlic, onion, and ginger in a large pot, which is heavy-bottomed and stir over medium to high heat. Keep stirring until the mixture turns fragrant or for about 3-5 minutes.

2. Add chopped carrot along with the pumpkin and keep stirring for the next 5-7 minutes, followed by adding marjoram, broth, bay leaves and the red lentils.

3. Boil the soup and simmer it gradually.

4. Once you have stirred in all spices as well as the tamari, allow the soup to stew for the next half hour, until carrots and pumpkins are delicate and tender.

5. Right before serving, add torn pieces of kale leaves cooked gently in the hot soup.

6. Adjust to taste with sea salt and ground pepper.

DAY 6

BAKED EGGS

/ SERVES 6 / PREPARATION TIME 5 MIN. / COOKINGTIME 30 MIN. /

INGREDIENTS

1	tbsp butter
6	eggs (medium to large)
1	tbsp ground black pepper (fresh)
¾	tbsp salt (for taste)
2	tbsp cream (whipped)
6	ramekins or custard cups (6 ounce each)

NUTRITION PER SERVING

CALORIES — 127   PROTEIN — 7.5   FIBER — 0

SUGARS — 2   FAT — 10.35

INSTRUCTIONS

1. Preheat the oven to 350°C.

2. Coat each of the 6 custard cups or the ramekins with ½ tbsp of butter.

3. Break an egg into each prepared custard cup or the ramekin.

4. Sprinkle the pepper and salt thoroughly over the eggs.

5. Combine each egg with the 1 tbsp of cream.

6. Keep each of the 6 ramekins or the custard cups in a baking dish (13x9 inch) and pour 1 and ¼ inches of hot water into the pan

7. Bake the mixture at 350°C for the next 30 minutes until the eggs are set.

TIP
Add Italian herbs to the baked eggs while serving and try with the lemon-pepper seasoning to add flavour to the recipe.

ROASTED DELIACTA SQUASH IN CHILE SAUCE

/ SERVES 4 / PREPARATION TIME 10 MIN. / COOKINGTIME 35 MIN. /

INGREDIENTS

1	finely halved, cored and sliced delicate squash (sliced in ½ inch semi circles)
3	completely dried Ancho, pasilla or guajillo chiles
2	cups of water
2	finely diced garlic cloves
2	crushed black peppercorns
½	tbsp of salt to taste
1	tbsp extra-virgin olive oil

NUTRITION PER SERVING

CALORIES — 40   PROTEIN — 1.3   FIBER — 1.3

SUGARS — 4.0   FAT — 0

INSTRUCTIONS

1. Keep the sliced delicata squash into a bowl while separately coming up with the chile sauce.

2. Remove the seeds and the stems of the chilies and heat them on medium to high heat in a skillet, in order to toast them.

3. Remove the chilies and place them in a pan along with the 2 cups of water and bring them to boil and let it sit for 15-20 minutes.

4. Drain them, but be careful in removing the water they've soaked in and put it aside.

5. Take the chilies and place in a blender along with the garlic, pepper, salt, and 1 to 1 ½ cups of the soaking liquid, while stirring the mixture until it becomes smooth and pure.

6. Mix olive oil in together with the sauce and introduce the chili sauce in with the squash.

7. Keep the squash out on a baking tray and bake at 375°F for about 15 to 20 minutes, while turning the squash over in the middle of the bake time.

OPEN FACED LOX SANDWICH

/ SERVES 1 / PREPARATION TIME 10 MIN. / COOKINGTIME 0 MIN. /

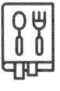

INGREDIENTS

1 slice pumpernickel bread
2 tbsp part-skim ricotta
4 oz. smoked salmon
2 tbsp capers
1½ tbsp minced onions

NUTRITION PER SERVING

CALORIES — 380   PROTEIN — 34   FIBER — 2
SUGARS — 1   FAT — 13

INSTRUCTIONS

1. Place the ingredients layer by layer in the order mentioned above.

2. Starting from the 1 sliced pumpernickel bread, place the following ingredients one by one to form a fine open-faced lox sandwich.

BREAKFAST BURRITO

/ SERVES 6 / PREPARATION TIME 10 MIN. / COOKINGTIME 5 HOURS /

INGREDIENTS

Finely cooked and drained pork sausage roll –
1 Pound
Finely cooked and crumbled bacon strips, ½ pound
18   lightly beaten medium to large eggs
Couple of cups of frozen and shredded hash brown
thawed potatoes
1   finely chopped large onion
Condensed and undiluted cheddar cheese soup
(1 can (10-¾ ounces)
Finely chopped green chilies 1 can (4 unces)
1   tbsp garlic powder
½   tbsp pepper for taste
Couple of cups of shredded cheddar cheese
10   warm flour tortillas (10 inches)

NUTRITION PER SERVING

CALORIES — 390   PROTEIN — 21   FIBER — 11
SUGARS — 1   FAT — 25.1

INSTRUCTIONS

1. Combine the first nine ingredients in a large bowl.
2. Combine half of the egg mixture into a slow cooker coated with cooking spray, while topping with almost half of the cheese.
3. While you repeat the layers, continue to cook low for the next 5 hours or until the thermometer reads 160°.
4. Spoon 3/4th cup of the egg mixture across center of each tortilla.
5. Fold bottom and sides of tortilla over filling and roll up.

ROASTED BROCCOLI WITH BRUSSELS SPROUTS

/ SERVES 8 / PREPARATION TIME 5 MIN. / COOKINGTIME 20 MIN. /

INGREDIENTS

Broccoli florets (1 pound)

Brussels sprouts (½ pound)

2 tbsp extra virgin olive oil

Sea salt and pepper to taste

NUTRITION PER SERVING

CALORIES — 187.6   PROTEIN — 11.6   FIBER — 11.7

SUGARS — 3.3   FAT — 8.0

INSTRUCTIONS

1. Preheat the microwave oven to 400°F.

2. Combine the broccoli, Brussels sprouts and olive oil in a bowl and toast nicely to coat.

3. Spread the broccoli and Brussels sprouts on a uniform layer on a baking sheet if possible.

4. Sprinkle the mixture with salt and pepper, while keeping the baking sheet in oven and roast for the next 20 minutes or until you see the mixture is starting to turn brown a little.

SKILLET BEEF TAMALE

/ SERVES 5 / PREPARATION TIME 10 MIN. / COOKINGTIME 35 MIN. /

INGREDIENTS

1	pound lean ground beef (90% lean)
⅓	cup chopped sweet red pepper
⅓	cup chopped green pepper
2	cups salsa
¾	cup frozen corn
2	tbsp water
6	corn tortillas (6 inches), halved and cut into ½-inch strips
¾	cup shredded reduced-fat cheddar cheese
5	tbsp fat-free sour cream

NUTRITION PER SERVING

CALORIES — 329	PROTEIN — 5	FIBER — 6
SUGARS — 4.8	FAT — 11	

INSTRUCTIONS

1. Cook beef and peppers in a medium to large non-stick skillet which is finely coated with cooking spray, over medium heat for up to 10minutes or until beef doesn't remain pink in color and vegetables seem more tender, which leads to the beef breaking up into crumbles, eventually drain.

2. Boil the mixture while stirring in the salsa, corn and water. Also, stir in the tortilla strips. Slightly decrease the heat; simmer while it is covered, for the next 15 minutes until the tortillas are tender.

3. Gently add some cheese and continue cooking while keeping the skillet covered for the next 3 minutes or until the cheese starts to melt. Serve the delicious recipe with sour cream.

TIPS
For best results, use a cast-iron skillet, or substitute another oven-proof skillet with tall sides.

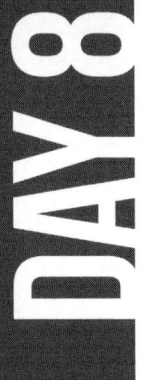

GREEN FRITTERS

/ SERVES 2 / PREPARATION TIME 15 MIN. / COOKINGTIME 15 MIN. /

INGREDIENTS

140g finely grated courgettes
3 medium eggs
85g finely chopped broccoli florets
3 tbsp gluten-free flour or rice flour
2 tbsp sunflower oil (for frying)
Small pack dill, roughly chopped

NUTRITION PER SERVING

CALORIES — 310   PROTEIN — 15   FIBER — 4
SUGARS — 2   FAT — 11

INSTRUCTIONS

1. Firmly squeeze the courgettes down, in order to remove any excess moisture.

2. Beat the eggs in a bowl, bring in the broccoli, courgettes and most of the dill, and combine them thoroughly well. Bring in the flour, mix them together again and season. In a non-stick frying pan, heat the oil and drop a medium serving spoon of the mixture in the pan followed by adding a couple of more spoonfuls of the mixture in order to have 2 fritters.

3. Heat over medium heat for 4 minutes or until it develops a golden brown color on one side and it gets solid enough for you to flip over.

4. Flip it over and allow it gain a golden complexion on the other side. Repeat to make one more fritter.

5. Spread the remaining dill over the fritters to serve.

BURRITO BOWL WITH CHIPOTLE BLACK BEANS

/ SERVES 2 / PREPARATION TIME 7 MIN. / COOKINGTIME 25 MIN. /

INGREDIENTS

125g basmati rice
400g can black beans, drained and rinsed
100g chopped curly kale

1 tbsp olive oil
2 garlic cloves, chopped
1 tbsp cider vinegar
1 tsp. honey
1 tbsp chipotle paste
1 avocado, halved and sliced
1 medium tomato, chopped
1 small red onion, chopped

NUTRITION PER SERVING

CALORIES — 340   PROTEIN — 17   FIBER — 10
SUGARS — 5   FAT — 9

INSTRUCTIONS

1. Cook the rice and leave it in the pan to keep warm.
2. Meanwhile in the frying pan, add the garlic and fry for 2 minutes over the heated oil until it turns golden in color.
3. Add the beans, vinegar, honey and chipotle.
4. Stir and let it warm for the next 2 minutes.
5. Boil the kale for a minute and then drain it.
6. Uniformly distribute the rice in between big shallow bowls and finely top them with the beans, kale, avocado, tomato and onion.
7. You are ready to serve with hot sauce, coriander and lime wedges.

CHICKEN VEGETABLE SKILLET

/ SERVES 2 / PREPARATION TIME 10 MIN. / COOKINGTIME 20 MIN. /

INGREDIENTS

2	tbsp seasoned breadcrumbs
½	pound boneless skinless chicken breast, cut into 1-inch strips
2	tsp canola oil, divided
1	small onion, chopped
½	cup sliced fresh carrot
1	small zucchini, sliced
1	small yellow summer squash, sliced
2	garlic cloves, minced
¼	tsp. pepper
⅛	tsp. salt
2	tbsp shredded cheese

NUTRITION PER SERVING

CALORIES — 259   PROTEIN — 5   FIBER — 3
SUGARS — 3.7   FAT — 10

INSTRUCTIONS

1. First and foremost, keep the breadcrumbs in a medium to large resalable plastic bag.

2. Gradually add the chicken and shake thoroughly to coat with the breadcrumbs.

3. Cook chicken in a large skillet coated with cooking spray, with 1 tsp oil, over medium to high heat or until the juices are evidently running.

4. Remove the mixture and ensure it remains warm.

5. Sauté onion and carrot in the same skillet, using the remaining oil until it turns crispy and tender.

6. Introduce the zucchini, garlic squash, pepper and salt and bring them to boil for another 5 minutes or until vegetables are tender.

7. Take the chicken back to pan and sprinkle with cheese.

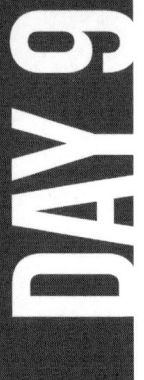

NUT, BUTTER, BANANA AND CHIA SEED TOAST

/ SERVES 4 / PREPARATION TIME 10 MIN. / COOKINGTIME 0 MIN. /

INGREDIENTS

Half cup of peanut butter
(natural only and creamy)
1 tbsp chia seeds
1 tbsp honey
8 slices of whole-grain bread
2 freshly ripe sliced bananas
Cinnamon and sea salt (for sprinkling)

NUTRITION PER SERVING

CALORIES — 337   PROTEIN — 13   FIBER — 0
SUGARS — 4.5FAT 14

INSTRUCTIONS

1. Stir together the peanut butter, chia seeds and honey, in a small bowl.

2. Spread nearly 2 tbsp of the above mixture on each of the four slices of bread.

3. Add a layer of sliced bananas on the top of the peanut butter's layer.

4. Sprinkle with cinnamon and sea salt.

5. Make a sandwich by placing the second slice of bread over the other

6. Divide in the diagonal half to eat instantly.

SALMON CUCMBER TARTARE

/ SERVES 2 / PREPARATION TIME 7 MIN. / COOKINGTIME 0 MIN. /

INGREDIENTS

3	oz. canned pink salmon, drained
1	tbsp capers
1	tsp. yellow mustard
2	tbsp plain low-fat yogurt
1	cucumber
	Dash salt
	Dash pepper

NUTRITION PER SERVING

CALORIES — 349   PROTEIN — 30   FIBER — 5

SUGARS — 1   FAT — 28

INSTRUCTIONS

1. Combine the first six ingredients in a fine proportion.

2. Halve the cucumber lengthwise and take out the mass to hollow it out.

3. Stuff the two hollowed halves with the salmon mixture to prepare your cucumber salmon boats and serve fresh.

ONE POT HAM AND PENNE SKILLET

/ SERVES 1 / PREPARATION TIME 5 MIN. / COOKINGTIME 15 MIN. /

 ## INGREDIENTS

1	tbsp olive oil
½	cup chopped yellow onion
3	cloves minced garlic
3	cup cubed fully cooked ham
½	tsp. dried parsley
½	tsp. dried basil
¼	tsp. dried oregano
¼	tsp. pepper
¼	tsp. red pepper flakes
3	cups chicken broth
2	cups 2% low FAT — milk
¼	cup flour
1	(16 oz.) penne noodles, uncooked
2	cups frozen peas, thawed
½	cup Parmesan cheese

NUTRITION PER SERVING

CALORIES — 430   PROTEIN — 21   FIBER — 5
SUGARS — 5   FAT — 17

 ## INSTRUCTIONS

1. Drop 1 tablespoon of olive oil in a medium to large skillet over medium heat.
2. Bring the onions and the ham to a boil until the onions turn translucent in shade.
3. Add the oregano, garlic, pepper, and parsley, basil, and red pepper flakes and cook the mixture for the next couple of minutes.
4. Stir milk, penne noodles and the flour in the broth and cook them for another 10 minutes.
5. Bring in the peas and cook the recipe for another five minutes or until the pasta seems to be completely cooked through and peas are warmer.
6. Gently sprinkle the Parmesan cheese on top of pasta to enjoy the recipe more.

DAY 10

AVOCADO TOAST WITH EGG

/ SERVES 6 / PREPARATION TIME 5 MIN. / COOKINGTIME 15 MIN. /

 ## INGREDIENTS

1   pitted and peeled avocado
1   can of diced tomatoes & green chillies (drained)
1   tbsp lime juice
½   tbsp divided salt
No-stick cooking spray
6   eggs
⅓   cup onion cream cheese spread
6   slices of toasted oval shaped whole grain bread
⅛   tbsp ground black pepper for taste

 ## NUTRITION PER SERVING

CALORIES — 350   PROTEIN — 11.1   FIBER — 8.5
SUGARS — 2   FAT — 20

INSTRUCTIONS

1. Finely mash the avocado's in a small to medium bowl and stir them add drained tomatoes lime juice and quarter tea spoon of salt and set it aside.

2. Spray the skillet with cooking spray and hear it over medium heat.

3. Introduce the eggs; cover the mixture and cook it for another 7 minutes or until the required doneness is reached.

4. Simultaneously, finely spread over the cream cheese on the bread slices. You could top them with the avocado mixture and eggs. Sprinkle the remaining salt and pepper on eggs and serve fresh.

SPICY TUNA AND COTTAGE CHEESE

/ SERVES 1 / PREPARATION TIME 15 MIN. / COOKINGTIME 1 HOUR /

INGREDIENTS

1   can of drained tuna (250 grams)
Finely chopped ½ red chilli
1   sliced spring onion
Few halved tomatoes
½   small bunch of chopped coriander
1   medium-sized potato (jacket)
Cottage cheese (150 grams and low fat)

NUTRITION PER SERVING

CALORIES — 350   PROTEIN — 44   FIBER — 3
SUGARS — 4   FAT — 5

INSTRUCTIONS

1. Preheat the oven to 180F.
2. Prick the potato many a times using a fork and place onto the hottest shelf in the oven.
3. Bake for approximately an hour until it is tender inside.
4. Next, combine the tuna with chili, spring onion, cherry tomatoes and coriander.
5. Split open the medium sized jacket potato and fill it using the tuna mix and cottage cheese.

TIP
You can use any combination of these shredded cheeses instead of the cheese blend in this recipe: Parmesan, mozzarella, Asiago, Fontina or Romano.

FRESH CORN AND TOMATO FETTUCCINE

/ SERVES 4 / PREPARATION TIME 5 MIN. / COOKINGTIME 5 MIN. /

INGREDIENTS

8	ounces uncooked whole-wheat fettuccine
2	medium ears sweet corn, husks removed
2	tsp plus
2	tbsp olive oil, divided
½	cup chopped sweet red pepper
4	green onions, chopped
2	medium tomatoes, chopped
½	tsp. salt
½	tsp. pepper
1	cup crumbled feta cheese
2	tbsp minced fresh parsley

NUTRITION PER SERVING

CALORIES — 370   PROTEIN — 17   FIBER — 10

SUGARS — 3.8   FAT — 15

INSTRUCTIONS

1. Cook fettuccine in a Dutch made oven, as per the guidelines written on the packing, carefully adding the corn during the last few minutes of cooking the fettuccine.

2. Simultaneously, heat 2 tsp oil over medium-high heat in a small to medium sized skillet.

3. Add cook and stir the red pepper and green onions until they appear tender.

4. Drain the pasta along with the corn and shift the pasta into a much larger bowl.

5. Cool down the corn and remove it from the cob and mix it with the pasta.

6. Now add tomatoes, oil, pepper and not to forget the pepper mixture.

7. Gently toss to combine the mixture in a finer proportion and sprinkle with cheese to serve.

SCRAMBLED EGGS MUFFINS

/ SERVES 3 / PREPARATION TIME 10 MIN. / COOKINGTIME 20 MIN. /

INGREDIENTS

½	pound pork sausage in bulk
12	eggs
½	cup onion (chopped)
½	cup green bell pepper (chopped)
½	tsp salt (to taste)
¼	tsp ground black pepper (to taste)
¼	tsp garlic powder
½	cup shredded Cheddar cheese

NUTRITION PER SERVING

CALORIES — 49.9   PROTEIN — 4.9   FIBER — 0.2

SUGARS — 0.9   FAT — 2.4

INSTRUCTIONS

1. Stir the eggs in with the sausage while heating the large pan over medium to high heat.

2. Continue to cook and stir until your sausage turns crumbly, with a complete brown shade. This should take around 10 to 15 minutes.

3. In the meantime, beat the 12 eggs in a medium to large bowl.

4. Stir in onion, green pepper, salt, pepper, and garlic powder and mix these ingredients in the sausage and Cheddar cheese.

TIP
Aluminium foil work wonders to keep the recipe healthy and moist while ensuring that it is being cooked uniformly. It keeps leftovers fresh, and makes clean up easy.

GREEN CLUB SANDWICH

/ SERVES 1 / PREPARATION TIME 10 MIN. / COOKINGTIME 0 MIN. /

INGREDIENTS

3 fine slices of the wholegrain toast
3 tbsp of all readymade humus
1 stoned and sliced small avocado worth 100g
Few rocket leaves
8-12 finely sliced cherry tomatoes

NUTRITION PER SERVING

CALORIES — 453   PROTEIN — 18   FIBER — 12
SUGARS — 4   FAT — 35

INSTRUCTIONS

1. Toast the whole-grain bread and evenly spread the humus onto each side of the slice.

2. On one slice of the bread, keep half the avocado, rocket and tomato.

3. Sprinkle with pepper and cover with the other slice.

4. Put on the rest of the avocado, rocket and tomato while sprinkling again and topping with the third slice.

PEANUT CHICKEN STIR FRY RECIPE

/ SERVES 6 / PREPARATION TIME 15 MIN. / COOKINGTIME 15 MIN. /

INGREDIENTS

8	ounces uncooked thick rice noodles
⅓	cup water
¼	cup reduced-sodium soy sauce
¼	cup peanut butter
4½	tsp honey
1	tablespoon lemon juice
2	garlic cloves, minced
½	tsp crushed red pepper flakes
1	pound boneless skinless chicken breasts cut into ½-inch strips
2	tbsp canola oil, divided
1	bunch broccoli, cut into florets
½	cup shredded carrot

NUTRITION PER SERVING

CALORIES — 361   PROTEIN — 24   FIBER — 5

SUGARS — 4   FAT — 13

INSTRUCTIONS

1. Cook the noodles as per the guidelines written on the package.

2. Simultaneously, mix the water, honey, peanut butter, soy sauce, lemon juice, pepper flakes in a small to medium skillet and keep it aside.

3. Carefully stir and fry the chicken in a large skillet, in 1-tablespoon oil unless and until the chicken is no longer pink in color.

4. Keep it aside and ensure that it remains warm. Take broccoli and carrots and stir-fry them in the remaining oil for up to 6 minutes and until vegetables turn crispy and tender.

5. Meanwhile, stir the sauce mixture and mix together the sauce and chicken within the skillet.

6. Place the chicken back in the skillet.

7. Carefully drain the noodles and toss them with the chicken mixture to boost the taste of the recipe.

CHOCOLATE OATMEAL RECIPE

/ SERVES 2 / PREPARATION TIME 10 MIN. / COOKINGTIME 10 MIN. /

INGREDIENTS

1	cup almond milk
½	cup oats rolled nicely
½	tbsp cinnamon
¼	tbsp ground nutmeg
¼	tbsp ground clove
1	tbsp dark chocolate (unsweetened)
½	cup of pureed pumpkin (plain)
2	tbsp honey
1	tbsp dried cherries
1	tbsp almonds (silvered)

NUTRITION PER SERVING

CALORIES — 136   PROTEIN — 3   FIBER — 4

SUGARS — 1.4   FAT — 2

INSTRUCTIONS

1. Bring the milk to boil in a saucepot. Introduce oats and allow it to simmer. Continue to cook as you stir the mixture frequently, until the oats are all cooked and the liquid is completely absorbed.

2. Quickly add the cinnamon, nutmeg, clove, and chocolate until the chocolate is completely melted and gets distributed throughout.

3. Mix in the pumpkin and honey, while stirring often till it mixes thoroughly with the oatmeal.

4. Top with the beautiful cherries while placing spoons into bowls. You are ready to serve and enjoy the dish.

TIP
Cookie dough can be covered and refrigerated for up to 24 hours before baking. If it becomes too firm, let it stand at room temperature for 30 minutes.

RED LANTEL AND SWEET POTATO PATE

/ SERVES 4 / PREPARATION TIME 20 MIN. / COOKINGTIME 20 MIN. /

INGREDIENTS

1½ tbsp olive oil
½ finely chopped onion
1 tsp. smoked paprika
1 finely peeled and diced small sweet potato
140g red lentils
500ml low-sodium vegetable stock
3 thyme leaves (chopped)
1 tsp. red wine vinegar
Vegetable sticks and pitta bread to serve

NUTRITION PER SERVING

CALORIES — 200   PROTEIN — 9   FIBER — 3
SUGARS — 5   FAT — 5

INSTRUCTIONS

1. Heat the oil in a large pan while slowly adding on the onion. Cook gently until it turns tender and golden in color.

2. Bring in the paprika and cook it for the next 2 minutes. Additionally add the sweet potato, lentils, thyme and stock and bring the mixture to boil, while cooking for the next 20 minutes or till the point the potatoes and lentils are softer and tender.

3. Put in some vinegar and seasoning, and thoroughly mash the mixture till you get your favorite texture.

4. Chill it for the next 1 hour and drizzle with olive oil.

5. Sprinkle the mixture with the thyme sprigs and serve with pitta bread and the vegetable sticks.

CHICKEN THIGHS WITH SHALLOTS AND SPINACH

/ SERVES 6 / PREPARATION TIME 10 MIN. / COOKINGTIME 30 MIN. /

 ## INGREDIENTS

6   boneless skinless chicken thighs
       (about 1½ pounds)
½   tsp seasoned salt
½   tsp. pepper
1½ tsp olive oil
4   shallots, thinly sliced
⅓   cup white wine or reduced-sodium
       chicken broth
1   package (10 ounces) fresh spinach, trimmed
¼   tsp. salt
¼   cup fat-free sour cream

 ## NUTRITION PER SERVING

CALORIES — 225   PROTEIN — 24   FIBER — 1
SUGARS — 2   FAT — 10

INSTRUCTIONS

1. Bring in the chicken and sprinkle it with seasoned salt and pepper.

2. Heat oil over medium to high heat, within a large non-sticky skillet finely coated with the cooking oil or the spray.

3. Mix in the chicken to the skillet while you cook it for the next 6 minutes on either sides or until the thermometer gives a reading of 170°.

4. Remove the chicken from the pan while ensuring that it remains warm yet fresh.

5. Cook and stir shallots in the same pan until they become soft and tender. Then mix wine into the mixture and bring it to boil.

6. Keep cooking till the wine decreases by half. Merge in the spinach and salt as per your requirements, as you cook and stir the ingredients until the spinach starts to wilt.

7. Stir in sour cream and serve with chicken, and you are ready to begin.

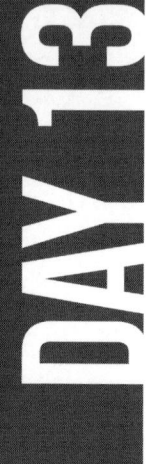

HONEY OATMEAL SQUARES

/ SERVES 25 / PREPARATION TIME 5 MIN. / COOKINGTIME 15 MIN. /

INGREDIENTS

½   cup margarine

½   tbsp almonds or **½** tbsp of vanilla extract

½   cup honey

2   cups rolled oats (packed)

NUTRITION PER SERVING

CALORIES — 210   PROTEIN — 6   FIBER — 5

SUGARS — 4.6   FAT — 2.5

INSTRUCTIONS

1. Melt down the margarine and combine it with the extract and the honey.
2. Introduce oats to the mixture and mix it well.
3. Press the apparatus into an ideal sized baking pan (8 inches).
4. Bake the apparatus for 15 minutes at 350°F or till the point bubbles show up and turn golden brown in colour.
5. Cool it down and cut into 25 equal squares.

TIP
Freeze individually wrapped bars up to 1 month; thaw at room temperature before enjoying.

HEALTHY CHICKPEA SOUP

/ SERVES 4 / PREPARATION TIME 5 MIN. / COOKINGTIME 20 MIN. /

INGREDIENTS

1	tbsp olive oil
1	medium chopped onion
2	chopped celery sticks
2	tsp. ground cumin
600ml	hot vegetable stock
400g	can of plum tomatoes with garlic
400g	can chickpeas (rinsed and drained)
100g	frozen broad beans zest and juice
½	lemons (Large)
	Handful of coriander or parsley and handful of flatbread (for serving)

NUTRITION PER SERVING

CALORIES — 148   PROTEIN — 9   FIBER — 6
SUGARS — 1.7   FAT — 5

INSTRUCTIONS

1. In a large saucepan, heat the oil followed by frying the onion and celery gently for at least 10 minutes or until it becomes tender, while stirring regularly.

2. Add the cumin and keep frying for another one minute. Increase the heat, and add the stock, tomatoes and chickpeas, in addition to a fine grind of black pepper and bring it to boil for another 10 minutes.

3. Add broad beans and lemon juice, and cook for a couple of minutes more.

4. Top with a drizzle of lemon zest and chopped herbs to serve with flatbread.

CRUMB COATED RED SNAPPER

/ SERVES 4 / PREPARATION TIME 15 MIN. / COOKINGTIME 10 MIN. /

INGREDIENTS

½	cup dry breadcrumbs
2	tbsp grated Parmesan cheese
1	tsp. lemon-pepper seasoning
¼	tsp. salt
4	red snapper fillets (6 ounces each)
2	tbsp olive oil

NUTRITION PER SERVING

CALORIES — 288   PROTEIN — 36   FIBER — 0

SUGARS — 1   FAT — 10

INSTRUCTIONS

1. Combine the lemon pepper, breadcrumbs, cheese, and salt within a shallow bowl as you add fillets, one after the other, and gradually turn to coat.

2. Take a heavy skillet and heat it over medium heat.

3. Now, gradually cook the fillets in oil, in a certain number of batches, for up to 5 minutes on either side or till the point the fish is easy to flake with the fork.

Day 14 — Breakfast

SOUTHWESTERN TOFU SCRAMBLE

/ SERVES 4 / PREPARATION TIME 10 MIN. / COOKINGTIME 20 MIN. /

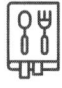

INGREDIENTS

3 tbsp of canola oil (divided)
1 Firm water-packed tofu packet (14 ounce) rinsed and crumbled
1½ tbsp of chilli powder
1 tbsp of ground cumin
½ tbsp salt (divided)
1 diced and small zucchini
¾ cup of thawed frozen corn
4 sliced scallions
¼ cup freshly chopped cilantro
½ cup shredded cheese
½ cup salsa (prepared)

NUTRITION PER SERVING

CALORIES — 202   PROTEIN — 13   FIBER — 3
SUGARS — 1   FAT — 12

INSTRUCTIONS

1. In a large non-stick skillet, heat 1½ tsp oil.
2. Now add tofu, chilli powder, cumin and ¼ tsp salt while cooking and stirring simultaneously till the tofu begins to develop a brown shade (shall take up to 6 minutes).
3. Transfer the apparatus to the bowl.
4. Now mix the 1½ tsp of oil to the pan and mix zucchini, corn, scallions and the remaining ¼ tsp salt. Keep cooking and stirring until, the vegetables become delicate, which shall take up to 3 minutes.
5. Meanwhile, come back to the tofu in the pan and keep cooking and stirring it until it is thoroughly heated for about 2 minutes.
6. Remove the apparatus from the heat and keep stirring the cheese until it melts down.
7. Sprinkle each serving with 2 tbsp of salsa and a tablespoon of cilantro.

SPICY AVOCADO WRAPS

/ SERVES 2 / PREPARATION TIME 8 MIN. / COOKINGTIME 5 MIN. /

INGREDIENTS

½	x 300g pack of chicken styled pieces
½	lime
½	tsp. mild chilli powder
1	finely chopped garlic clove
1	tsp. olive oil
2	seeded wraps
1	halved and stoned avocado
1	roasted and chopped red pepper

NUTRITION PER SERVING

CALORIES — 403   PROTEIN — 29   FIBER — 5
SUGARS — 2   FAT — 16

INSTRUCTIONS

1. Mix the vegetarian chicken-style pieces with the lime juice, chili powder and the garlic.

2. Meanwhile, in a non-stick frying pan, heat the oil followed by frying the pieces for a couple of minutes, as you heat them over the flame to slightly char them.

3. Do not allow to dry them out. Then, squash one half of an avocado onto each wrap. Introduce the peppers to the pan and warm them thoroughly.

4. Fill the wraps with the chicken-style pieces while rolling them up and eating them with your fingers.

TIP
To blanch the asparagus and pea pods, plunge them into boiling water for 10 to 15 seconds or until they turn bright green.

CHICKEN VEGETABLE SKILLET

/ SERVES 2 / PREPARATION TIME 10 MIN. / COOKINGTIME 20 MIN. /

INGREDIENTS

2 tbsp seasoned breadcrumbs

½ pound boneless skinless chicken breast, cut into 1-inch strips

2 tsp canola oil, divided 1 small onion, chopped

½ cup sliced fresh carrot 1 small zucchini, sliced

1 small yellow summer squash, sliced

2 garlic cloves, minced

¼ tsp pepper

⅛ tsp. salt

2 tbsp shredded Asiago cheese

NUTRITION PER SERVING

CALORIES — 259   PROTEIN — 28   FIBER — 3

SUGARS — 4.6   FAT — 10

INSTRUCTIONS

1. Place bread crumbs in a large resalable plastic bag.
2. Add chicken and shake to coat. In a large skillet coated with cooking spray, cook chicken in 1 tsp oil over medium heat until juices run clear.
3. Remove and keep warm. In the same skillet, sauté onion and carrot in remaining oil until crisp-tender.
4. Add the zucchini, squash, garlic, pepper and salt; sauté 4-5 minutes longer or until vegetables are tender.
5. Return chicken to pan; sprinkle with cheese.

BANANA PEANUT BUTTER CHIA PUDDING

/ SERVES 6 / PREPARATION TIME 15 MIN. / COOKINGTIME 0 MIN. /

INGREDIENTS

2	freshly ripe bananas
1½	cups of low FAT — milk
½	cup peanut butter
3	tbsp of chia seeds

NUTRITION PER SERVING

CALORIES — 258   PROTEIN — 12   FIBER — 14

SUGARS — 14.3   FAT — 7.6

INSTRUCTIONS

1. Pour the two bananas, milk and the creamy peanut butter in a blender.

2. Now, shift the mixture to a medium sized bowl and keep stirring the mixture while adding the chia seeds.

3. Next, cover the mixture with a plastic wrap and leave it to refrigerate for another 4 hours or overnight.

4. Stir the mixture thoroughly before serving it.

TIP
The recipe could be easily stored in an airtight container and be re-frigerated for up to 1 week.

TUNA RICE SALAD

/ SERVES 8 / PREPARATION TIME 15 MIN. / COOKINGTIME 15 MIN. /

INGREDIENTS

900g cooked rice
400g tuna in spring-water
200g defrosted frozen petits pois
2 red peppers
3 finely chopped tomatoes
5 finely sliced spring onions
Flat-leaf parsley, chopped
Green olives (roughly chopped)
4 tbsp mayonnaise
2 tbsp extra-virgin olive oil
1 lemon

NUTRITION PER SERVING

CALORIES — 370
SUGARS — 3

PROTEIN — 14.11
FAT — 16.31

FIBER — 3.6

INSTRUCTIONS

1. Break the cooked rice up in a large mixing bowl.
2. Add the tuna and mix in the peas, peppers, tomatoes, spring onions, parsley and olives.
3. Stir in the mayonnaise, lemon juice and olive oil and season to taste.
4. Use cling film to cover the bowl.
5. You are ready to serve and enjoy.

QUINOA, BROCCOLI AND CHEDDAR GRATIN

/ SERVES 4 / PREPARATION TIME 10 MIN. / COOKINGTIME 25 MIN. /

INGREDIENTS

1	tbsp olive oil, plus more for greasing
1	large leek, thinly sliced
1	large shallot, thinly sliced
2	garlic cloves, minced
½	tsp. fresh thyme leaves (or ¼ tsp dried)
½	tsp. salt
1¼	pounds broccoli, cut into small florets
3	cups cooked quinoa (from 1 cup uncooked)
1	large egg, beaten
1½	cups sharp cheddar cheese, shredded

NUTRITION PER SERVING

CALORIES — 41   PROTEIN — 2.1   FIBER — 0.5
SUGARS — 2   FAT — 2.1

INSTRUCTIONS

1. Preheat the oven to 400°.
2. Drop some oil in a large cast-iron skillet and bring it to boil. If not a skillet then you could even use a warm casserole dish.
3. Grease a large lidded saucepan.
4. Boil the leek and the shallots over medium heat until they turn soft and tendered or for about 5 minutes.
5. Add the garlic, salt and thyme while you continue cooking for another 1 minute.
6. Add the broccoli and cook as you keep stirring it occasionally until it turns bright green in color or for a couple of minutes.
7. Add a quarter cup of water and cook until the liquid has considerably decreased and the broccoli has got tender, which should not take more than 3 minutes.
8. Take it off the heat and stir in the quinoa, 1 cup of cheese and eggs. Shift them to the prepared dish and formalize an even layer.
9. Top the recipe with the cheese that remains.
10. For best results, you could bake until the cheese develops a brown shade or for about 20 minutes.

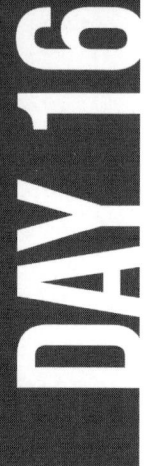
SPINACH AND CHEDDAR MICRO-WAVE QUICHE

/ SERVES 1 / PREPARATION TIME 5 MIN. / COOKINGTIME 3 MIN. /

INGREDIENTS

½ cup finely chopped spinach
(frozen, thawed and properly drained)

1 egg

⅓ Cup of low FAT — milk

⅓ Cup of cheddar cheese (shredded)

1 chopped slice of bacon (cooked)
Salt and pepper just to taste

NUTRITION PER SERVING

CALORIES — 231   PROTEIN — 11   FIBER — 1
SUGARS — 3.1   FAT — 16.1

INSTRUCTIONS

1. Keep the freshly chopped spinach in a mug and add a couple of tsp of water. Cover the apparatus with a paper towel, while keeping the microwave on high temperature for almost one full minute.

2. Take the apparatus out of the microwave and drain the excess water or liquid from the spinach thoroughly.

3. Next, break the egg within the mug, adding it to the spinach and milk, complimented by cheese and bacon. (Additionally add some salt and pepper as per your taste)

4. Mix the ingredients until it combines perfectly well. Cover closely with a paper towel and microwave on high temperature for 3 minutes.

SPICY ROOT AND LENTIL CASSEROLE

/ SERVES 4 / PREPARATION TIME 5 MIN. / COOKINGTIME 40 MIN. /

INGREDIENTS

2	tbsp sunflower or vegetable oil
1	chopped onion
2	finely crushed garlic clove
700g	peeled and chunked potatoes
4	thickly sliced carrots
2	thickly sliced parsnip
2	tbsp curry paste or powder
1	¾ pints vegetable stock
100g	red lentils
	Roughly chopped fresh coriander
	Low FAT — yogurt
	Low FAT — bread to serve

NUTRITION PER SERVING

CALORIES — 378   PROTEIN — 14   FIBER — 10
SUGARS — 1   FAT — 9

INSTRUCTIONS

1. Cook the onion and the garlic over the medium to high heat for up to 4 minutes or until it becomes tender, while stirring it occasionally. Meanwhile heat the oil in a large pan.

2. Add the potatoes, carrots and parsnips. Switch the heat on and cook for another 6-7 minutes, while continuing to stir, until the vegetables turn a golden color.

3. Stir in the curry paste or powder, and add the remaining stock and boil the mixture.

4. Turn down the heat and add the lentils. Cover the pan and simmer again for 15-20 minutes until the lentils and vegetables are soft and the sauce has gained thickness.

5. Stir in the coriander, stir it and heat for a minute.

6. Top it using the yogurt and coriander.

7. You are ready to serve it with naan bread.

LEMONY COLLARD GREEN PASTA

/ SERVES 1 / PREPARATION TIME 5 MIN. / COOKINGTIME 15 MIN. /

INGREDIENTS

8 ounces fresh collard greens
(about 10 big leaves)

⅓ or more of a package of whole wheat
thin spaghetti or "spaghetti"

3 tbsp pine nuts olive oil (the good stuff)

2 small cloves garlic, pressed
Big pinch red pepper flakes
Sea salt and black pepper

1 ounce Parmesan cheese

½ or more of a lemon, cut into wedges

NUTRITION PER SERVING

CALORIES — 475   PROTEIN — 20   FIBER — 15
SUGARS — 1   FAT — 29

INSTRUCTIONS

1. Boil the salted water within a large sized pot and cook the pasta as per the guidelines.

2. Drain the water, just ensuring a little bit of cooking water, and keep it one side

3. Be careful in cutting out the center rib of the collard green as you pile some greens in order to roll them into cigar-kind of shape.

4. The rolls must be kept as slim as possible (⅛" to ¼").

5. Chop the greens to make sure that the strands are not as long.

6. Toast the pine nuts on a heavy-bottomed 12" skillet heated over medium heat until they start turning golden and fragrant.

7. Take them out of the skillet and return the skillet to medium heat and drop in a tablespoon or two of the olive oil.

8. Throw in a few of the red pepper flakes together with the garlic and stir. Toss in all of your collard greens, once the oil is hot enough to simmer.

9. Shower the greens with salt while you stir often, and boil the greens for about three minutes.

10. Take the greens away from the pan and scoop them into the pasta pot to toss with another drizzle of olive oil.

11. Top with pine nuts and Parmesan shavings and serve warm.

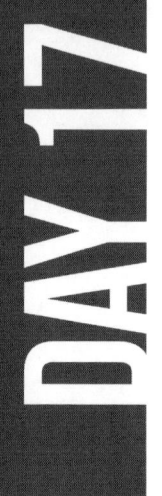

QUINOA AND CHIA PORIDDGE

/ SERVES 1 / PREPARATION TIME 10 MIN. / COOKINGTIME 10 MIN. /

INGREDIENTS

¾	cup cooked quinoa (cooked)
1	tbsp chia seeds
½	cup almond or coconut milk (low fat)
½	tbsp of ground cinnamon (for taste)
¼	tbsp ground cardamom (it is optional)
	Some amount of sea salt (for taste)
	Seasonal fruit, rice, yoghurt, walnuts and some extra cinnamon

NUTRITION PER SERVING

CALORIES — 290   PROTEIN — 9   FIBER — 0
SUGARS — 3   FAT — 15

INSTRUCTIONS

1. Add all the chia seeds, spices, low FAT — milk and the quinoa in a small to medium pan and bring it to simmer over medium heat.

2. Keep the gentle simmering while you continue to stir occasionally for the next 5 minutes, or till the milk is completely absorbed by the mixture.

3. You could add extra milk if your porridge gets too dry.

4. Serve the freshly prepared porridge with yoghurt, walnuts, and fruit, a pinch of syrup complimented by a sprinkle of extra cinnamon.

RISOTTO WITH BACON PEACE

/ SERVES 4 / PREPARATION TIME 5 MIN. / COOKINGTIME 45 MIN. /

INGREDIENTS

1 onion
6 finely chopped rashers streaky bacon
300g risotto rice
1 hot vegetable
100g frozen pea

NUTRITION PER SERVING

CALORIES — 315   PROTEIN — 5   FIBER — 0
SUGARS — 3   FAT — 15

INSTRUCTIONS

1. Finely chop the onion.
2. Meanwhile, heat the 2 tbsp of olive oil along with a knob of butter in the pan.
3. Add the onions and fry them until they turn light brown in color (about 7 minutes).
4. Add the bacon in the pan and fry for the next 5 minutes, until it begins to get crisp.
5. Add the rice and stock to the mixture and boil them altogether.
6. Stir the mixture thoroughly, and then reduce the heat and continue to heat it over medium heat for 15-20 minutes or until the rice becomes soft and tender.
7. Add the peas and stir the mixture while adding a little salt and pepper and continue to cook the mixture for a further 3 minutes.
8. You could serve the lunch sprinkled with freshly grated Parmesan and black pepper.

TIP
Serve with additional freshly grated Parmesan cheese and freshly ground black pepper.

BAKED CHICKPEA AND TOMATO EGG PLANT

/ SERVES 3 / PREPARATION TIME 15 MIN. / COOKINGTIME 45 MIN. /

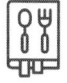

INGREDIENTS

3 small or medium eggplants
(round shaped are best for this recipe)
3 tbsp extra virgin olive oil
1 large onion, sliced thin across the grain
2 to **4** garlic cloves (to taste),
Minced **3** tomatoes, seeded and diced
1 sprig rosemary
1 (15-ounce) can chickpeas, drained
Salt and pepper to taste.

NUTRITION PER SERVING

CALORIES — 200   PROTEIN — 9   FIBER — 10.5
SUGARS — 5.1   FAT — 4.6

INSTRUCTIONS

1. Chop eggplants in halves and scoop out the bottom flesh, using a knife.

2. Keep aside the other halves and keep the smaller ones for later part of the procedure.

3. Preheat the oven to 400°F (200°C).

4. In a large, heavy skillet, heat 2 tbsp olive oil over medium heat.

5. Add the onion and cook while stirring often, until they turn tender or for about 2 minutes.

6. Add the garlic and salt. Keep cooking and stirring, until the garlic gains a fragrance, or for about a minute.

7. Add the diced tomatoes, salt to taste and sprig of rosemary.

8. Bring the mixture to a boil and stir often, for at least 5 minutes.

9. Introduce the freshly ground pepper, then taste and adjust seasoning.

10. Remove the rosemary sprig, while you keep stirring in the drained chickpeas.

11. Bring in the diced eggplant and keep cooking for another five minutes or until the sauce seems fragrant.

12. Stuff the eggplant cups using a spoon.

13. Transfer to a baking dish along with the eggplant's other halves, which were kept aside.

14. Sprinkle with olive oil and rosemary leaves. Next, Bake them in the oven for 20 – 30 minutes, or unless and until eggplant cups are softened.

15. You are ready to serve the delicious eggplants.

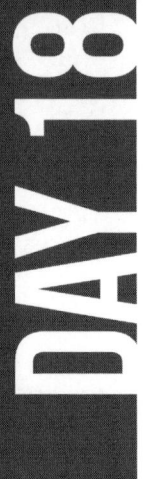

BREAKFAST TOMATO TOAST

/ SERVES 2 / PREPARATION TIME 10 MIN. / COOKINGTIME 0 MIN. /

INGREDIENTS

6-8 slices of your favorite bread

½ pound tomatoes chopped with a **¼** thickness

½ cup macadamia ricotta

¼ cup julienned shiso
Pinches of grain sea salt (For taste)

1 cup drained, rinsed and soaked raw macadamia nuts

1½ tbsp of nutritional yeast

2 tbsp apple cider vinegar

1½ tbsp fresh lime juice

2 tbsp white mellow paste

2 garlic cloves garlic

8-10 tbsp filtered water

¼ tbsp finely grained sea salt

NUTRITION PER SERVING

CALORIES — 228   PROTEIN — 5   FIBER — 0
SUGARS — 1   FAT — 0

 ## INSTRUCTIONS

1. Rinse the macadamia nuts and keep them together with nutritional yeast, vinegar, lemon juice, miso, garlic, 8 tbsp of water, and salt, in an upright blender with a high speed.

2. Let the apparatus blend on high for a minute, while you continue to scrap down the sides of the blender and gradually adding one tablespoon of water at one time until you reach a creamy constancy.

3. Add the salt and pepper as per your taste.

4. Cover the ricotta together with a cling wrap and refrigerate them together until you are ready to use it.

5. Sprinkle the toasted bread with macadamia ricotta along with the sliced tomatoes together with the julienned shiso, and a few pinches of black salt.

6. Cut the toast in halves and you are ready to serve.

HEALTHY STIR-FRIED RICE

/ SERVES 4 / PREPARATION TIME 10 MIN. / COOKINGTIME 10 MIN. /

INGREDIENTS

2	tbsp of sesame oil
½	shredded Chinese cabbage
1	carrot, which is chopped into matchsticks
1	small red capsicum (removed seeds and finely sliced)
3	cups of brown rice (cooked)
2	tbsp light soy sauce (tbsp)
2	tbsp and extra ketjap manis*
½	cup lightly toasted cashew nuts
6	thinly sliced spring onions

NUTRITION PER SERVING

CALORIES — 260	PROTEIN — 3	FIBER — 1
SUGARS — 1	FAT — 0	

INSTRUCTIONS

1. Heat the oil in a medium pan on high heat. Place in cabbage, carrot and capsicum while carefully stir-frying the mixture for the next 2 minutes.

2. Add rice and continue cooking the mixture for another 2 minutes. Add soy, ketjap manis, cashews and half the spring onions. Toss the mixture to combine it nicely.

3. Garnish with left over onions and drizzle with extra ketjap manis, in order to serve and enjoy the lunch recipe.

Day 18 — Dinner

PORK MEDAL-LIONS WITH SAUTEED APPLE

/ SERVES 4 / PREPARATION TIME 15 MIN. / COOKINGTIME 5 MIN. /

INGREDIENTS

2	tsp. cornstarch
⅔	cup reduced-sodium Chicken broth
¼	cup apple juice
1	tbsp butter
2	medium apples, thinly sliced
2	green onions, sliced
1	garlic clove, minced
¾	tsp dried thyme
½	tsp paprika
¼	tsp. salt
¼	tsp. pepper

1-pound pork tenderloin, cut into 1-inch slices

NUTRITION PER SERVING

CALORIES — 251   PROTEIN — 25   FIBER — 10
SUGARS — 3   FAT — 10

INSTRUCTIONS

1. Preheat the boiler. Mix cornstarch, broth and apple juice in a small bowl.
2. Heat butter over medium-high heat, in a nonstick skillet.
3. Bring in the apples, garlic and green onions; cook and stir the mixture for the next 2-3 minutes or until apples turn crispy and tender.
4. Finely stir the mixture and introduce it to the pan.
5. Boil the mixture while cooking and stirring it for another 1-2 minutes or until the mixture gains thickness.
6. Add the thyme, paprika, salt and pepper. Put the pork slices with a meat mallet to half inside.
7. Now, place the pork gently, on a broiler pan.
8. Broil 3 inches from heat 3-4 minutes on either side.
9. Let it stand firm for 5-10 minutes before you serve.

TIP
Make this dish lower in sodium by using reduced-sodium pig broth.

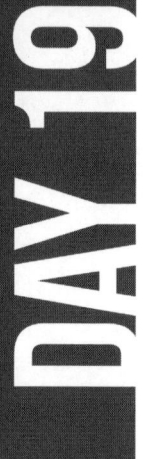

FRESH FRUIT SALAD

/ SERVES 1 / PREPARATION TIME 5 MIN. / COOKINGTIME 5 MIN. /

INGREDIENTS

2	cups of freshly sliced strawberries
2	cups of green seedless grapes, which are halved
1	small cantaloupe, which is cut into chunks
2	firmly sliced bananas
⅓	cups of completely fresh orange juice

NUTRITION PER SERVING

CALORIES — 75   PROTEIN — 0   FIBER — 1

SUGARS — 4   FAT — 0

INSTRUCTIONS

1. Combine all the fruits in a medium to large bowl.

2. Pour the juice carefully over the fruits and toss them nicely to coat.

3. Cover the apparatus and refrigerate it for at least 4 hours.

STUFFED SWEET PO-TATOES WITH BLACK BEANS AND AVOCADO

/ SERVES 1 / PREPARATION TIME 10 MIN. / COOKINGTIME 1 HOUR /

INGREDIENTS

	Sweet potato (small in size)
1	tbsp extra-virgin olive oil
1	finely chopped onion
1	finely minced clove garlic
1	cup finely chopped tomato
1	cup freshly rinsed and drained black beans
2	tbsp cheddar cheese (low fat)
½	cubed avocado
2	tbsp freshly chopped cilantro

NUTRITION PER SERVING

CALORIES — 1   PROTEIN — 5   FIBER — 5
SUGARS — 2   FAT — 8

INSTRUCTIONS

1. Preheat oven to 425°F. Peel the sweet potato.
2. Add the foil-lined baking sheet and bake it for 45 minutes or until it gets soft and tender.
3. In a pan, stir the onion and garlic in oil for about 5 minutes. Now, Add the tomatoes and cook the mixture for another 5 minutes. Smash ½ of the black beans while adding the smashed mixture and remaining whole beans to the frying pan.
4. Cook the mixture for another 3 minutes until the beans are completely heated.
5. Cut the potato in two halves half. Now carefully take out the potatoes' flesh into a bowl and mash.
6. Now, you are supposed to replace the mashed sweet potato with the skins.
7. Top with remaining bean mixture, cheddar cheese, avocado, and cilantro.

SPAGHETTI WITH WILTED GREENS AND WALNUT PARSLEY PESTO

/ SERVES 6 / PREPARATION TIME 5 MIN. / COOKINGTIME 20 MIN. /

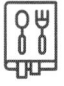

INGREDIENTS

1 (1-pound) box whole-wheat spaghetti
1 bunch Swiss chard, chopped
1 cup packed fresh flat-leaf parsley
½ cup packed fresh baby spinach
¼ cup walnuts, toasted
1 small clove garlic, peeled and chopped
2 tbsp plus 2 tsp olive oil
1 tsp finely grated lemon zest
½ tsp kosher salt, divided
½ tsp freshly ground black pepper, divided
6 large eggs

NUTRITION PER SERVING

CALORIES — 400   PROTEIN — 20   FIBER — 11
SUGARS — 2   FAT — 15

INSTRUCTIONS

1. Boil a large pot of water.
2. Now, Cook pasta as per the guidelines on the package.
3. Conserve a quarter cup of the pasta's cooking water.
4. Add the Swiss chard after 5 minutes of cooking the pasta and draining the extra water; leave the pasta and greens in the pot.
5. Meanwhile, mix parsley, spinach, garlic, 2 tbsp oil, walnuts, lemon zest, 1-tablespoon water, and quarter tsp each salt and pepper in a food processor; and ensure it is pulsed until it turns chunky.
6. Heat remaining olive oil in a large nonstick skillet, over medium-high heat. Crack batches of eggs into skillet and continue to cook until the whites become firm but the yolks still appear soft.
7. Dress up you egg recipe with remaining quarter tsp each salt and pepper.

CAULIFLOWER BREAKFAST MUFFINS

/ SERVES 3 / PREPARATION TIME 15 MIN. / COOKINGTIME 35 MIN. /

INGREDIENTS

2½	cup nicely diced cauliflower
1	tbsp ground flaxseed
2	finely beaten eggs
¼	tbsp table-salt (to taste)
⅛	tbsp pepper (to taste)
⅔	cup finely diced lean ham
2	cups of finely grated cheddar cheese
⅔	cup diced mushrooms
12	Jalapeno slices

NUTRITION PER SERVING

CALORIES — 118   PROTEIN — 9   FIBER — 1

SUGARS — 1   FAT — 8

INSTRUCTIONS

1. Preheat the oven to 375 degrees and keep the muffin in a 12 muffin-liners and spread with non-stick spray.

2. Combine all the ingredients in a medium sized mixing bowl, except the jalapenos.

3. Divide the ingredients evenly between the various muffin liners.

4. Place jalapeno slice on top of each muffin.

5. Bake the muffin for the next 30 minutes or until it turns brown in color.

RICE AND REFRIED BEANS

/ SERVES 4 / PREPARATION TIME 5 MIN. / COOKINGTIME 20 MIN. /

INGREDIENTS

2	tbsp olive oil
2	diced sausage links
1	cup long grain
	handful of uncooked white rice
2	finely crushed cloves of garlic
1	tbsp ground cumin
15	ounces of undrained canned diced tomatoes
15	ounces of drained canned Corn
2	cups of water
15	ounces of refried Beans
½	tbsp salsa

kosher salt (to taste)

hot sauce (to taste)

shredded Mexican Cheese (optional)

chopped cilantro (optional)

NUTRITION PER SERVING

CALORIES — 380   PROTEIN — 14   FIBER — 7
SUGARS — 1   FAT — 10.66

INSTRUCTIONS

1. Heat the oil thoroughly within a skillet over medium-high heat. Add the sausage and the rice together while stirring regularly for 4 minutes or until the rice increases in size and seems opaque enough and the sausage starts taking a brown color.

2. Add the garlic and cumin, and cook until it seems fragrant. Bring in tomatoes, corn, and water, while bringing this mixture to a boil and reduce the heat to medium.

3. Simmer for 15 minutes, and add the refried beans and salsa, while continuing to stir it.

4. Replace lid, and again simmer until the rice becomes soft tender.

5. Serve the recipe topped nicely with the shredded cheese, complimented with cilantro if desired.

CHICKEN BREASTS WITH SHAVED BRUSSELS SPROUTS

/ SERVES 4 / PREPARATION TIME 10 MIN. / COOKINGTIME 25 MIN. /

<u>INGREDIENTS</u>

2 (8-ounce) boneless, skinless chicken breast halves

¾ tsp kosher salt, divided

2 broccoli stems

2 tbsp olive oil

2 tbsp fresh lemon juice

¼ tsp freshly ground black pepper

3 cups thinly sliced Brussels sprouts (from 12 medium)

2 celery stalks, thinly sliced

¼ cup toasted hazelnuts

¼ cup fresh flat-leaf parsley, coarsely Chopped 1 ounce Parmesan cheese, coarsely grated

NUTRITION PER SERVING

CALORIES — 255.3   PROTEIN — 32   FIBER — 4.2
SUGARS — 3.2   FAT — 10.1

 ## INSTRUCTIONS

1. In a small saucepan, add the chicken and ½ a tsp of salt and cover with water; boiling the ingredients together. Instantly take them off the heat, cover the pan, and allow standing for the next 15 minutes.

2. Drain the chicken runs it under the cold water. When it cools completely; set it to one side.

3. In the meantime, utilize a vegetable peeler to remove the outer layer of broccoli stems, focusing the major attention on the long strips.

4. Whisk together oil, quarter tsp salt and pepper, lemon juice in a large nonstick skillet,

5. Add broccoli strips, celery, hazelnuts, Brussels sprouts, parsley, and reserved chicken to bowl with dressing; and toss together to coat firmly.

6. Top the dish with cheese.

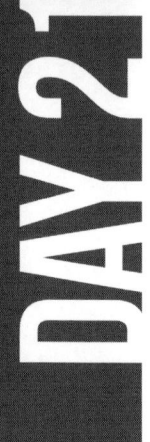

AVOCADO EGG-IN-A-HOLE

/ SERVES 4 / PREPARATION TIME 5 MIN. / COOKINGTIME 5 MIN. /

INGREDIENTS

1	fresh avocado
4	fine slices of bread
4	finely divided tbsp of butter
4	eggs
	Freshly ground black pepper and kosher salt
½	c. shredded sharp cheddar cheese
1	tbsp chopped chives

NUTRITION PER SERVING

CALORIES — 181   PROTEIN — 9   FIBER — 1.8
SUGARS — 2.8   FAT — 10.1

INSTRUCTIONS

1. Slice one fresh avocado in half and take out one large piece of flesh while keeping aside one half to cut it further into some large pieces, ensuring a hole in each of the slices.

2. Make a hole in the middle of each slice of bread, making sure that the hole is big enough to accommodate an avocado slice.

3. In a medium non-stick pan, melt 2 tbsp of butter over medium to high heat.

4. Add the two slices of bread to the pan and keep toasting on each side, for 2 minutes per side.

5. In the middle of each circle, break an egg and season it thoroughly with the salt and pepper.

6. Cover the pan and continue cooking for the next 3-5 minutes.

7. Add the cheese on top of each slice, cover it with a lid and cook to melt the cheese properly.

8. While garnishing with the chives, repeat the same process with the other ingredients.

SPROUT AND SPINACH SALAD

/ SERVES 8 / PREPARATION TIME 30 MIN. / COOKINGTIME 0 MIN. /

INGREDIENTS

1	freshly red onion (For dressing)
3	tbsp cider vinegar
1	tbsp honey
1	tbsp powdered mustard
½	cup extra-virgin olive oil
1	cherry tomato
4	cups of sprouts* (pea and lentil)
¾	pound of baby spinach.

NUTRITION PER SERVING

CALORIES — 227   PROTEIN — 4   FIBER — 2

SUGARS — 4   FAT — 7

INSTRUCTIONS

1. Cut the onion into half according to its length.
2. Chill an onion in the water for about half an hour by covering the onion with cold water kept in a bowl.
3. In the meantime, focus your attention on the dressing.
4. Whip the vinegar, mustard, salt and pepper altogether to taste.
5. Drain the onion thoroughly and dry it.
6. To serve , toss with onion, sprouts, spinach, and dressing.

BARLEY STUFFED POBLANOS

/ SERVES 1 / PREPARATION TIME 15 MIN. / COOKINGTIME 1 HOUR /

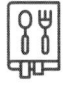 ## INGREDIENTS

3 tbsp olive oil, divided

1 large onion, diced

1½ cups barley, soaked overnight and drained

1 bunch kale, thick stems removed, leaves chopped

1⅛ tsp. chilli powder, divided

3 garlic cloves, minced

1 (28-ounce) can whole peeled tomatoes, crushed

¼ tsp kosher salt

6 large poblano peppers

2 ounces reduced-fat white cheddar, grated

3 slices (½ cup) reduced-fat Monterey Jack cheese, halved

½ cup crumbled pasteurized queso fresco

NUTRITION PER SERVING

CALORIES — 382   PROTEIN — 15   FIBER — 13
SUGARS — 1   FAT — 12

IINSTRUCTIONS

1. Heat 1 tablespoon oil over medium heat, in a large sauce-pan.

2. Add the onion and cook for 7 minutes until it gets tender.

3. Add barley and some water in order to cook it until barley is tender.

4. Until kale is wilted, stir kale and 1/8 tsp chili powder into barley and gradually mix in the cheddar.

5. Meanwhile, heat remaining oil over medium heat in a heavy pot.

6. Add the garlic and cook the mixture for another 3 minutes. Add tomatoes, remaining 1 tsp of chili powder, and salt; and boil the mixture. Decrease the heat and stir occasionally, till the sauce thickens. Finally, turn heat to lowest, cover it and set it to one side.

7. Heat the broiler in advance and slice off stems from peppers to ensure a broad hole for stuffing. Carefully remove membranes and seeds, using a small knife.

8. Using the mixture of barley, stuff peppers return the stem ends to top of peppers.

9. Keep in a large, broiler-proof baking dish; keep broiling till the peppers are charred and tender.

10. Add tomato sauce to the pan surrounded by the peppers. Carefully cover each pepper with half slice of the Monterey jack. Broil for another 2 minutes or until cheese melts

11. Finally transfer the peppers to plates drizzled with sauce; and top each with one tsp of queso fresco.

TIPS
For the best results, use leftover mashed potatoes, mashed potatoes from a box or pouch, or purchase refrigerated mashed potatoes.

CONCLUSION

CONGRATULATIONS!

Whether you chose the 21 or 10-day meal plan, you have suc-
cessfully completed a challenging but vitally important step
in eradicating "bad" sugar from your diet and reintroduc-
ing healthy, whole foods containing "Good" sugar into your
eating regime. At this point, your body has been running on
clean, consistent and even energy for days on end. You are
no longer relying on the "quick fix" of empty added sugar
calories. Gone are those all too brief energy spikes and ac-
companying crashes, requiring more and even more "bad"
sugar. You are feeling more rested, vigorous and happy and
more than likely, eating and drinking less than you have
in quite some time! Hopefully you have enjoyed the meals
from the plans in this book, trying new foods and adding
them to your favorites. The time you have spent preparing
these healthy, balanced recipes has resulted in improved
nutrition and energy, more than making up for so-called
"convenience" foods that rob you of your health!

If you are in need of motivation to continue this healthy life-
style, please take a moment and look at yourself in a
mirror. Now think back to the person you were mere days
or weeks ago: List the differences on a piece of paper and
stick it on your refrigerator as visual inspiration should
you feel like you miss some processed, sugary laden food
from your past. Is it really worth it? Is there something you
could do or accomplish or enjoy rather than backtracking
and risking your health and well-being?

Remember, life is a work in progress. If you do occasionally give
in to temptation or are fooled by a "Bad" sugar choice,
simply chalk it up to experience and move on. Don't pun-
ish yourself by repeating the mistake. Reward yourself with
a healthy, delicious whole food choice and celebrate your
success!

FREE DOWNLOAD

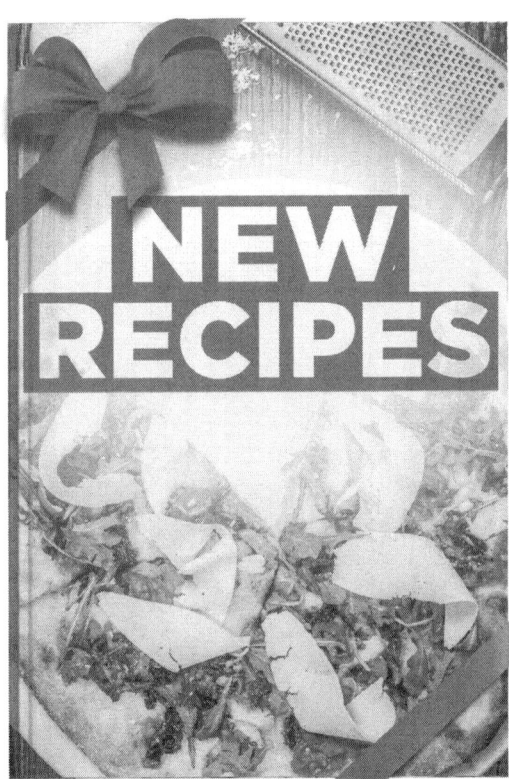

YOUR FREE GIFT!
GET MORE FREE RECIPES IN 1 CLICK!

GET YOUR FREE RECIPES HERE:

www.frenchnumber.net/detox21

All information is intended only to help you cooperate with your doctor, in your efforts toward desirable weight levels and health. Only your doctor can determine what is right for you. In addition to regular check ups and medical supervision, from your doctor, before starting any other weight loss program, you should consult with your personal physician.

Disclaimer and Terms of Use: Effort has been made to ensure that the information in this book is accurate and complete, however, the author and the publisher do not warrant the accuracy of the information, text and graphics contained within the book due to the rapidly changing nature of science, research, known and unknown facts and internet. The Author and the publisher do not hold any responsibility for errors, omissions or contrary interpretation of the subject matter herein. This book is presented solely for motivational and informational purposes only.

Presented by French Number Publishing
French Number Publishing is an independent publishing house head-quartered in Paris, France with offices in North America, Europe, and Asia.
FN№ is committed to connect the most promising writers to readers from all around the world. Together we aim to explore the most challenging issues on a large variety of topics that are of interest to the modern society.

Printed in Great Britain
by Amazon